JOKES MEN ON TOP

JOE KING

Strathearn Publishing

Strathearn Publishing
PO Box 44, Slough, Berkshire, SL1 4YN

Trade Distribution by W. Foulsham & Co. Ltd, The Publishing House, Bennetts Close, Cippenham, Slough, Berkshire, SL1 5AP, England

ISBN 0-572-02818-0

Printed in Great Britain by Cox & Wyman Ltd, Reading, Berkshire

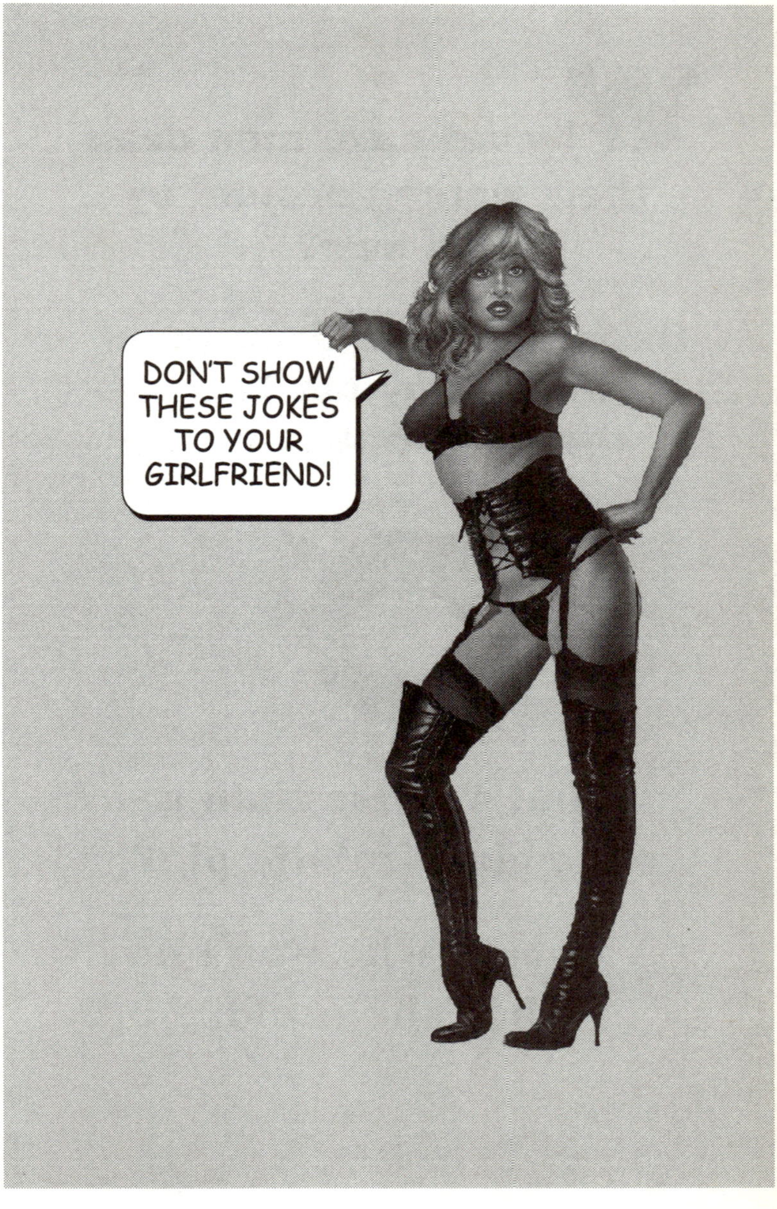
DON'T SHOW THESE JOKES TO YOUR GIRLFRIEND!

Why did cave men drag their women around by the hair?

Because if you drag them around by the feet they fill up with dirt.

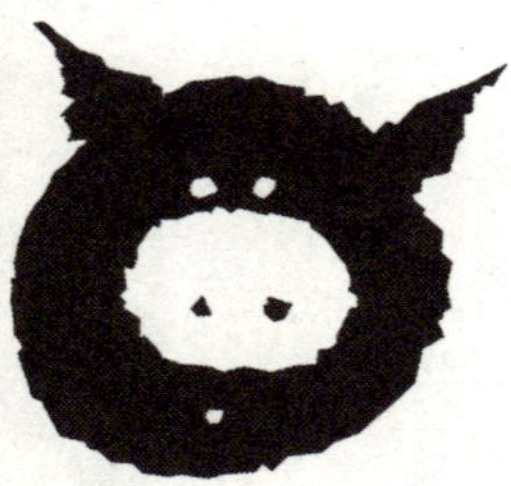

What's worse than a male chauvinistic pig?

A woman who won't do what she's told.

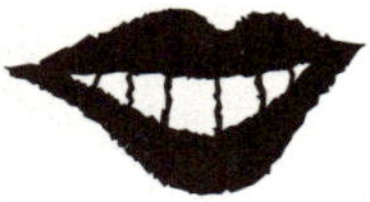

Why did God give men
PENISES?

So we'd always have
at least one way to
shut a woman up.

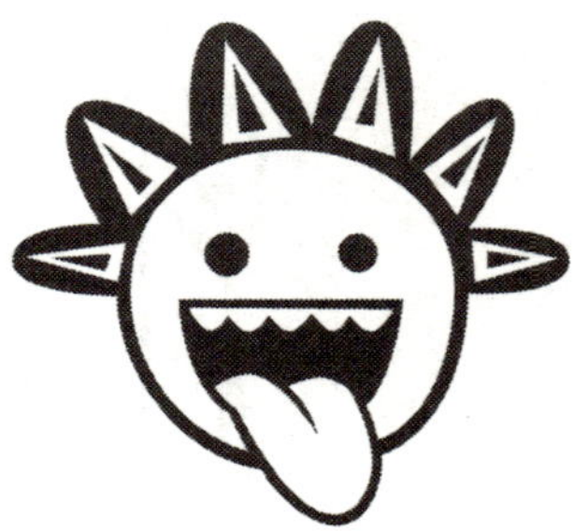

How do you know God meant men to eat pussy?

Why else would he make it look like a taco?

WHAT'S THE DIFFERENCE BETWEEN YOUR SALARY AND YOUR DICK?

YOU DON'T HAVE TO BEG A WOMAN TO BLOW YOUR SALARY.

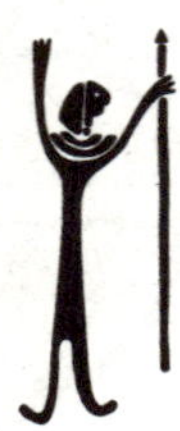

What's six inches long, two inches wide, and drives women wild?

Money.

A couple are staying in a hotel and annoyed to find they have twin beds. After a romantic dinner, they retire to bed but the man doesn't want to sleep.

'Come over to my bed, sweetheart,' he says to her. 'I'm seriously horny for you, you sexy woman.'

So the woman gets out of her bed to go to her husband's bed, but in the dark she trips on the rug and falls on her face.

'Oh, darling, are you all right?' the man asks in a concerned voice.

The woman gets up and climbs into the man's bed. The two have passionate sex and afterwards the woman rolls out.

As she returns to her bed, however, she catches her foot on the rug and falls flat on her face. The man turns over to go to sleep and says, 'Clumsy bitch'.

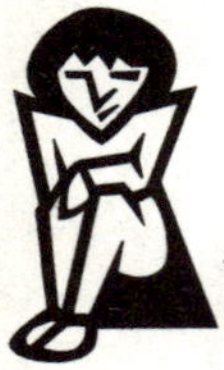

What's it called when a woman is paralysed from the waist down?

Marriage.

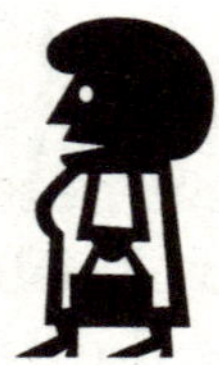

What's the most active muscle in a female?

The penis.

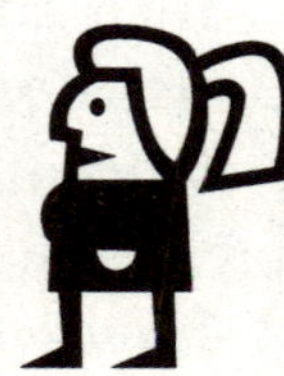

Why do men die before their wives?

They want to.

Why is a woman like a dog turd?

The older it is, the easier it is to pick up.

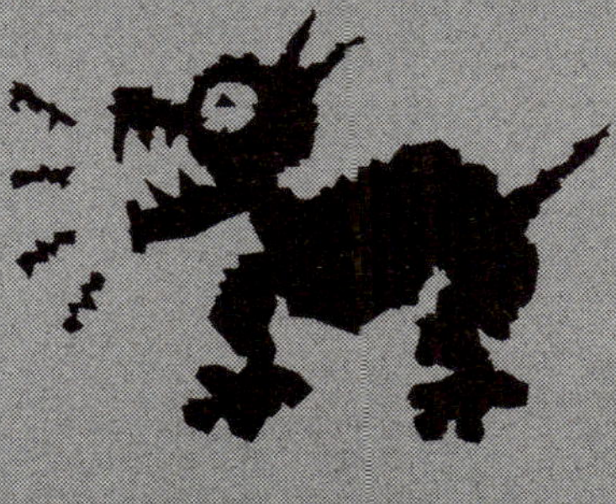

Ten things not to say when having sex

1. A little rug burn never hurt anyone.
2. I really hate women who think sex means something.
3. It's nice being in bed with a woman I don't have to inflate.
4. You're good enough to do this for a living.
5. And to think I was really trying to pick up your friend.
6. Do you accept Visa?
7. I was so horny tonight I could have shagged a horse!
8. They're not biscuit crumbs, it's just a rash.
9. And to think, I didn't even have to buy you dinner.
10. You can cook too, right?

Why did God make man first?

He didn't want to have a woman looking over his shoulder.

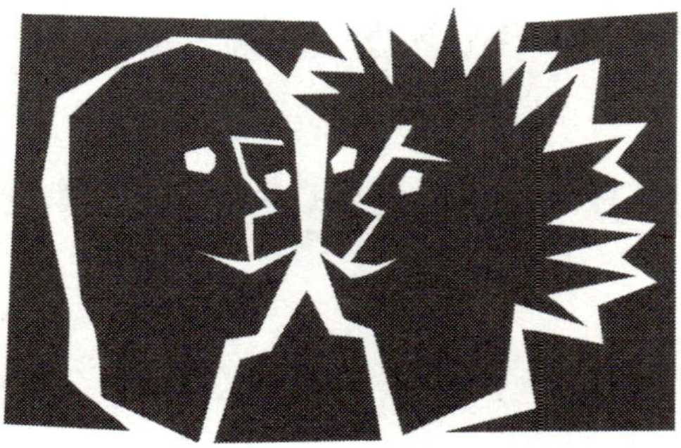

Why do women close their eyes during sex?

They can't stand seeing a man having a good time.

What do you call a woman who can suck an orange through a garden hose?

Darling.

How do you make a woman scream twice?

Fuck her up the arse, then wipe your dick on the curtains.

Chat-up lines to avoid

1 How do you like your eggs: fried, scrambled or fertilised?

2 If you and I were squirrels, I could bust a nut in your hole.

3 If your right leg was Christmas and your left leg was Easter, could I meet you between the holidays?

4 My love for you is like diarrhoea – I just can't hold it in.

5 Why don't we play lion and lion tamer? You hold your mouth open and I'll give you the meat.

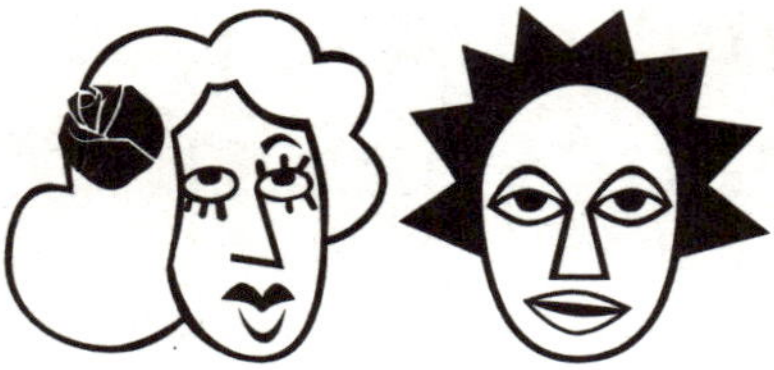

If you are having sex with two women and one more woman walks in, what do you have?

Divorce proceedings.

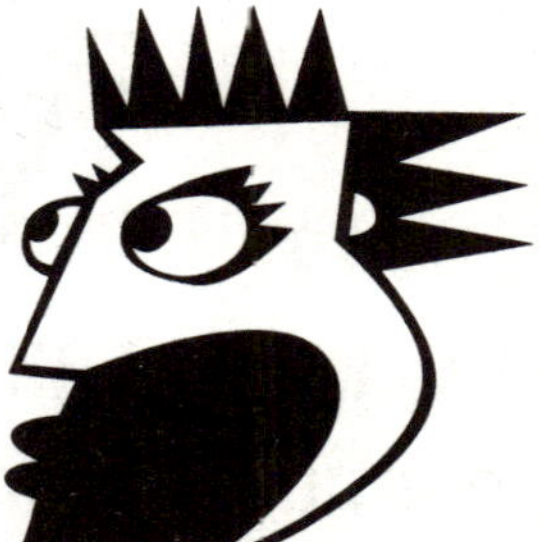

Why do men pass gas more than women?

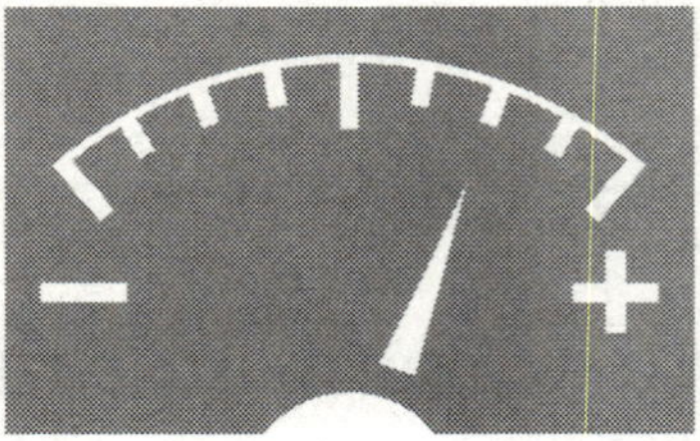

Because women won't shut up long enough to build up pressure.

What's the difference between a pregnant woman and a light bulb?

You can unscrew a light bulb.

If your wife keeps coming out of the kitchen to nag you, what have you done wrong?

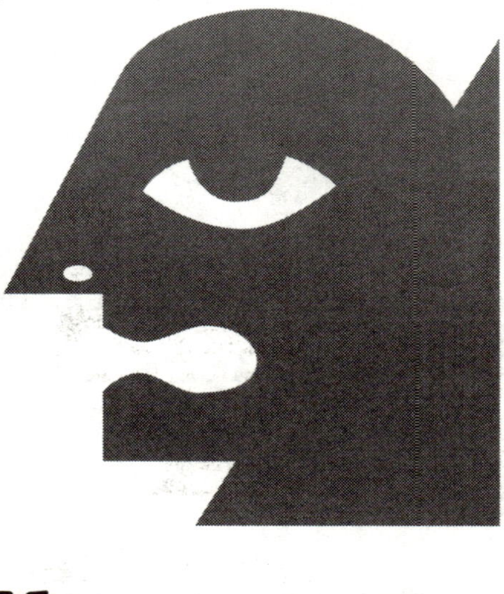

Made her chain too long.

WHY DID THE ARMY SEND SO MANY WOMEN WITH PMS TO THE GULF WAR?

THEY FOUGHT LIKE ANIMALS AND RETAINED WATER FOR FOUR DAYS.

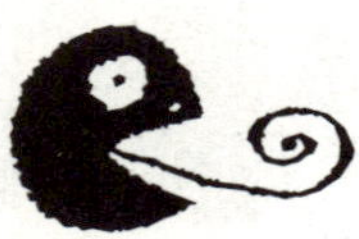

HOW CAN YOU TELL IF A WOMAN REALLY LIKES ORAL SEX?

SHE LIFTS UP HER SKIRT EVERY TIME SOMEONE YAWNS.

Why is a laundry a bad place to pick up women?

Because a woman who can't afford a washing machine will never be able to support you.

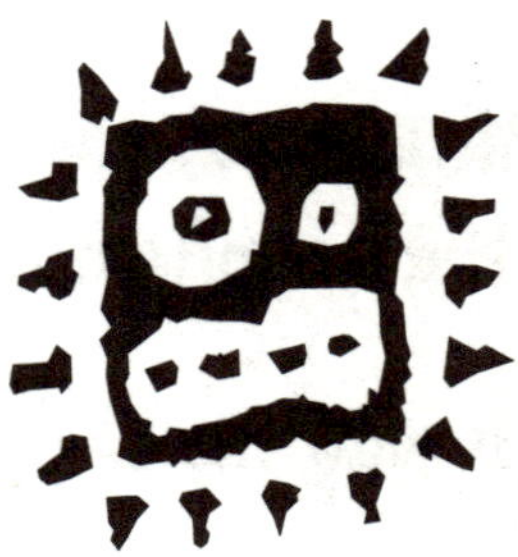

What's love?

The delusion that one woman is different from another.

Ten things you'll never hear a woman say

1 Could our relationship be more physical?

2 Go ahead and leave the seat up.

3 I think hairy butts are really sexy.

4 Hey, get a whiff of that one.

5 Please don't throw that old T-shirt away, the holes in the armpits are just too cute.

6 This diamond is way too big.

7 I won't even put my lips on that thing unless I get to swallow.

8 Wow, it really is 14 inches!

9 Does this make my bum look too small?

10 I'm wrong; you must be right again.

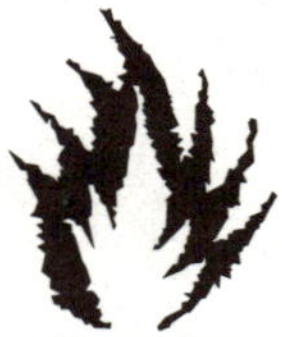

WHAT SHOULD YOU DO IF YOUR GIRLFRIEND STARTS SMOKING?

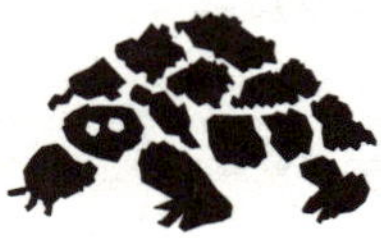

SLOW DOWN.

AND POSSIBLY USE A LUBRICANT.

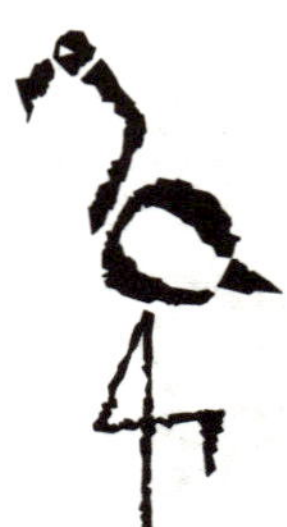

Did you hear about the new all-female delivery service?

It's called UPMS– they deliver whenever the hell they feel like it.

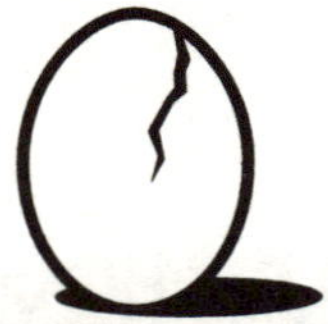

WHY DID GOD CREATE LESBIANS?

So feminists wouldn't breed.

?

What's the best thing about a blow job?

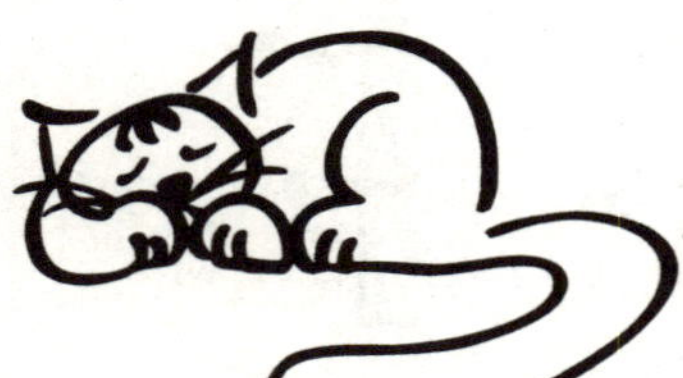

Ten minutes of silence.

Terry was digging his garden when two hearses drove slowly by, followed by a man walking solemnly along with a dog, and then about 200 men in single file.

Intrigued, Bill went up to the man following the second hearse and asked him who was in the first hearse.

'My wife,' the man replied.

'I'm sorry,' said Terry. 'What happened to her?'

'My dog bit her and she died.'

Terry then asked the man who was in the second hearse.

'My mother-in-law,' the man replied. 'My dog bit her and she died as well.'

Bill thought about this for a moment, then asked the man, 'Can I borrow your dog?'

To which the man replied, 'Get in line.'

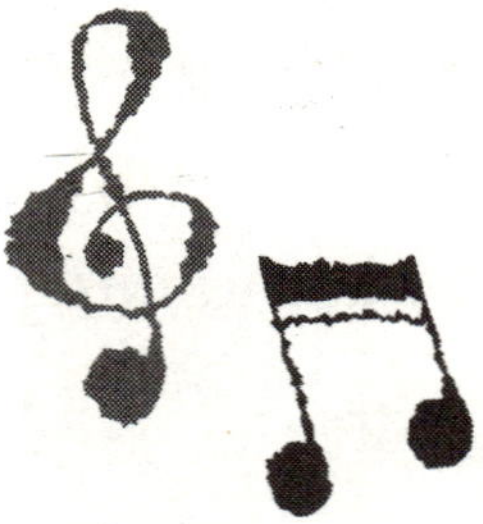

What is making love?

It's what a woman does while a man is screwing her.

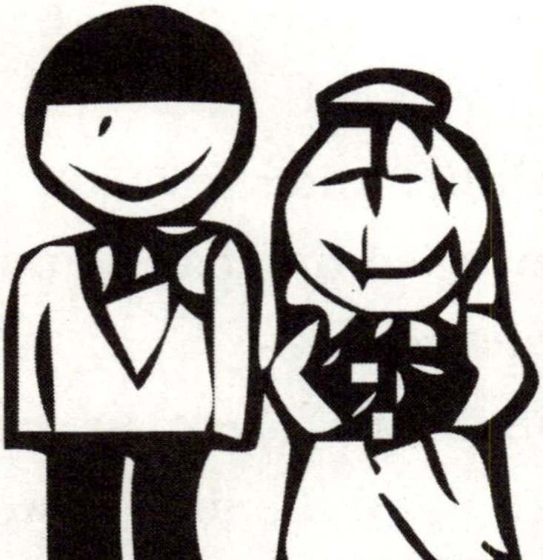

What do you call a woman who has lost 95 per cent of her intelligence?

Divorced.

Evening classes for women

Man management: discovering how the rubbish can wait until after the game.

Controlling communication: learning when to hang up the telephone.

The undiscovered side of banking: making deposits.

Personal space: leaving enough room in the bathroom cupboard for your partner's toothbrush.

What he really wants: is buying the right razor blades so difficult?

Retail management: you really can shop in less than four hours.

Gaining five pounds vs. the collapse of the market economy: a study in contrast.

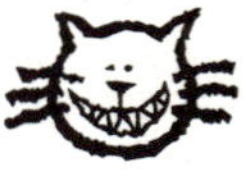

Why is a drugs officer like a male stud?

They are both crack investigators.

Why are women like rocks?

Because you skip the flat ones.

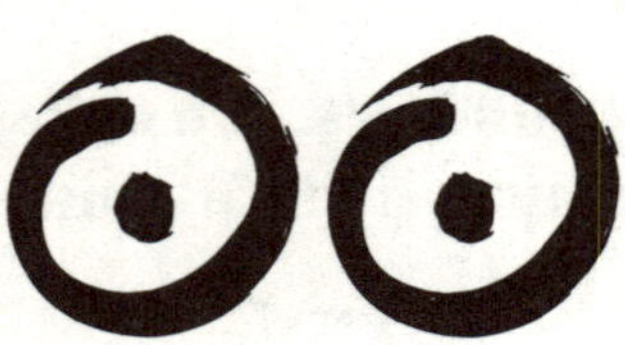

It's good to be a man because...

Your mates can be trusted never try to trap you with, 'Notice anything different?'

You get extra credit for the slightest act of thoughtfulness.

You can open your own jars.

You can make a telephone call in less than a minute.

Grey hair and wrinkles add character.

Same work ... more pay.

If you are 34 and single, nobody notices.

Car mechanics tell you the truth.

You don't have to shave below your neck.

Three pairs of shoes are more than enough.

You are unable to see wrinkles in your clothes.

You can do your Christmas shopping for 10 relatives on 24 December in 45 minutes.

If your wife drives you to drink...
... get her to drop you off at the pub.

Pete came home unexpectedly from a business trip to find his wife in the arms of his best friend.

'My God!' he shouted. 'I'm married to her so I HAVE to. But why you?'

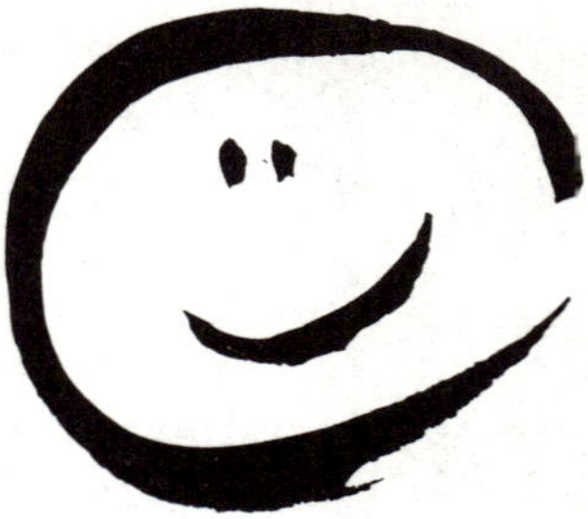

A man rushed into his house and shouted to his wife:

'Lucy, pack your bags. I've just won the jackpot on the lotto!'

'Oh, how exciting!' she replied. 'Shall I pack for warm weather or cold?'

'I don't care. Just as long as you're out of the house by noon!'

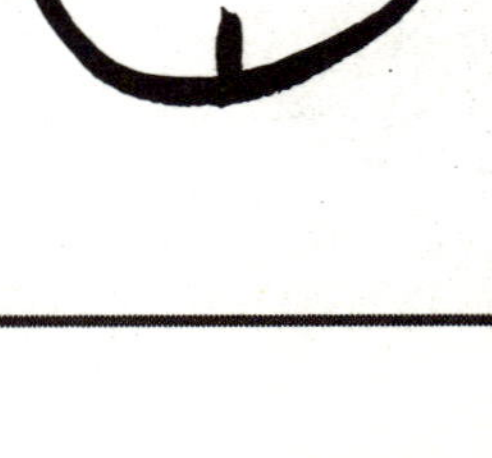

A man was sitting in the very best seats for the Cup Final, and the man next to him noticed there was an empty seat on the other side.

'Can you believe someone actually paid for that seat and didn't come to the match?' he said.

'Actually that's my wife's seat,' the man replied. 'We bought these tickets months ago, but my wife passed away so I came alone.'

'I'm sorry to hear that,' replied the first man. 'But why didn't you give the ticket to a family member or friend?'

'Oh, they're all at the funeral.'

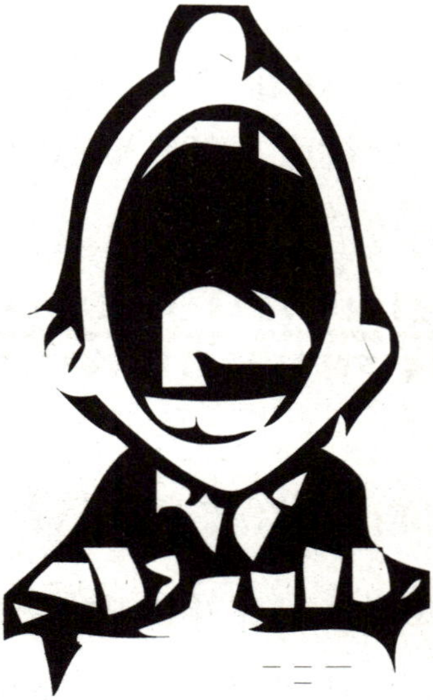

Why is e-mail like a man's dick?

It was created to transmit information vital to the survival of the species ... but most people use it just for fun.

Why are women like carpets?

Because if you lay them right the first time, you can walk all over them for the rest of your life.

A Man's Guide to Answering Questions No. 1

What are you thinking about?

Inappropriate answers:

(a) Sex (with other women).
(b) Football.
(c) How fat you are.
(d) How much prettier she is than you.
(e) How I would spend the insurance money if you died.
(f) If I wanted you to know what I was thinking, I would be talking to you.

Proper answer:

I'm sorry if I've been pensive, dear. I was just reflecting on what a warm, thoughtful, caring, intelligent woman you are, and how lucky I am to have met you.

'It's no good - I can't feel a thing,' she said. 'Your dick's too small.'

'Oh?' he replied. 'Perhaps that's because I'm playing in a cathedral.'

'My mother-in-law's an angel.'

'Lucky you. Mine's not dead yet.'

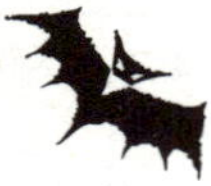

A Man's Guide to Answering Questions No. 2

Do I look fat?

Inappropriate answers:

(a) Compared to what?

(b) I wouldn't call you fat, but you're not exactly thin.

(c) A little extra weight looks good on you.

(d) I've seen fatter.

(e) Could you repeat the question? I was just thinking about how I would spend the insurance money if you died.

Proper answer:

Of course not!

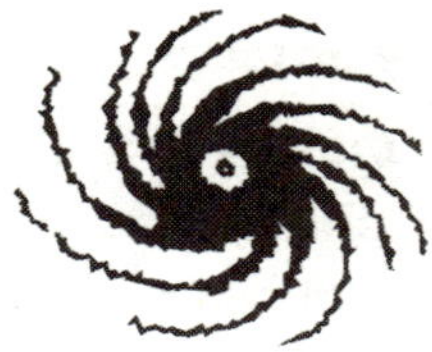

Why is a woman like a hurricane?

Because she starts out wet and wild, but when she goes she takes half your house.

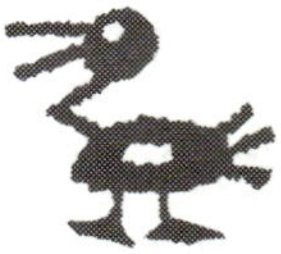

What's the difference between your wife and your job?

After five years your job will still suck.

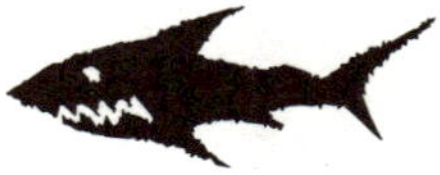

A Man's Guide to Answering Questions No. 3

Do you love me?

Inappropriate answers:

(a) Would it make you feel better if I said yes?

(b) Oh yeah, shit-loads.

(c) That depends on what you mean by love.

(d) Does it matter?

(e) Who, me?

Proper answer:

Yes. (Or if you feel a more detailed answer is in order) Yes, dear.

I bought my mother-in-law a lovely chair for her birthday....
but they won't let me plug it in.

How can you tell a woman is wearing tights?

Her ankles swell up when she farts.

A Man's Guide to Answering Questions No. 4

Do you think she is prettier than me?

Inappropriate answers:

(a) Not prettier, but definitely thinner.

(b) Yes, but you have a better personality.

(c) Not as pretty as you when you were her age.

(d) Define pretty.

(e) Could you repeat the question?
I was just thinking about how I would spend the insurance money if you died.

Proper answer:

Of course not!

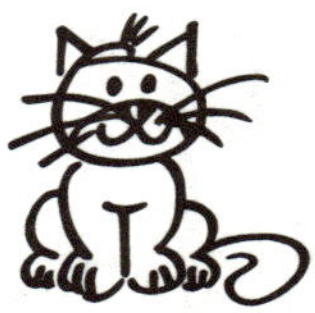

Why is a prostitute like a chicken farmer?

They both raise cocks for a living.

Why do women have two holes?

So when they get drunk you can carry them like a six-pack.

Why do female skydivers wear tampons?

So they won't whistle on the way down.

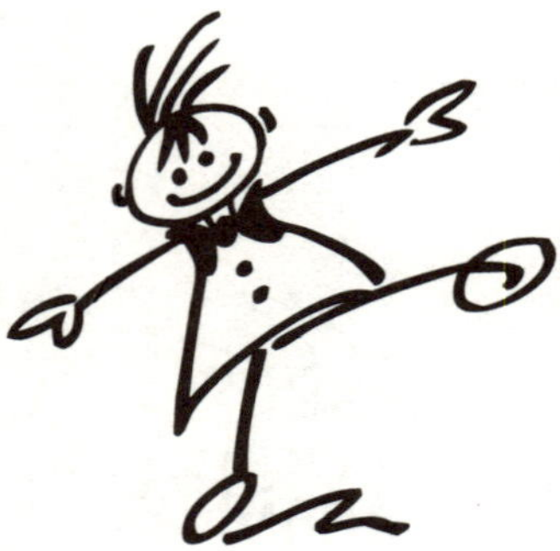

What two things in the air can make a woman pregnant?

Her legs.

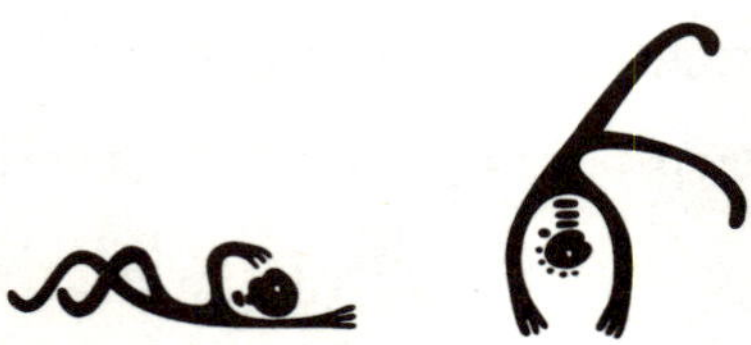

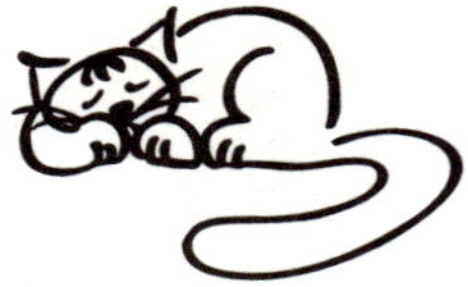

What do you call that useless piece of skin around a pussy?

A woman.

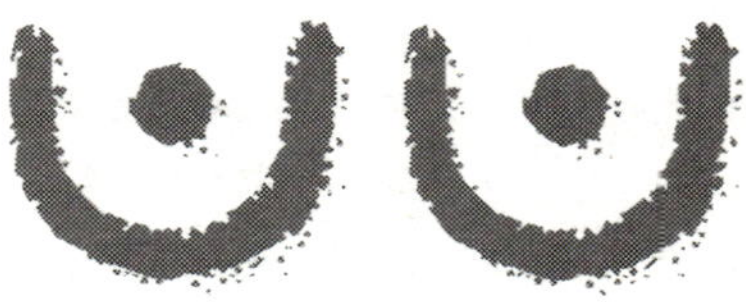

What are the small bumps around a woman's nipples for?

It's Braille for 'suck here'.

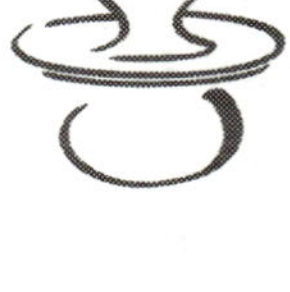

A Man's Guide to Women's English

Yes.	= No.
No.	= Yes.
Maybe.	= No.
I'm sorry.	= You'll be sorry.
We need.	= I want.
It's your decision.	= The correct decision should be obvious by now.
Do whatever you want.	= You'll pay for this later.
We need to talk.	= I need to complain.
Sure go ahead.	= I don't want you to.
You're so manly.	= You need a shave, and you sweat a lot.
I'm not upset.	= Of course I'm upset, you moron!
I heard a noise.	= I noticed you were almost asleep.
This kitchen is so inconvenient.	= I want a new house.
Be romantic - turn out the lights.	= I have flabby thighs.
Do you love me?	= I'm going to ask for something expensive.
How much do you love me?	= I did something today you're going to hate.
I'll be ready in a minute.	= Kick off your shoes and find a good game on TV.
You have to learn to communicate	= Just agree with me.
Are you listening to me!?	= (Too late, you're dead.)

Why are women like screen doors?

Once they get banged a few times, they loosen up.

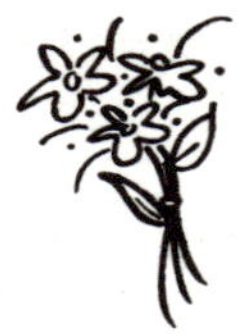

This day holds a lot of meaning for me.

It was on this day two years ago that I lost my dear wife and children.

I'll never forget that game of cards...

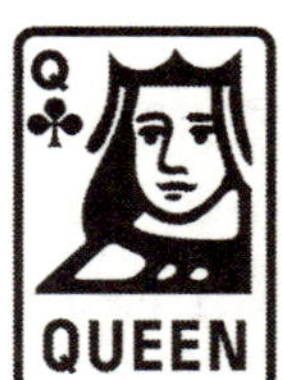

How can you tell which is the head nurse?

She's one with the dirty knees.

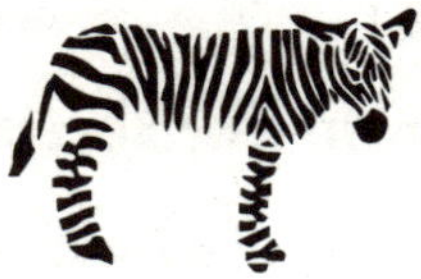

What is a zebra?

26 sizes larger than an A bra.

When God created Adam, it wasn't long before he started complaining that he was all alone in the Garden of Eden and he was lonely.

So God said, 'Okay, I'll make you a companion, a beautiful creature who'll cook and clean for you. She will be able to converse intelligently on any subject, and never ever complain or argue.'

'That sounds great,' Adam replied.

'The only thing is,' God said, 'it will cost you an arm and a leg.'

'Damn, that's expensive!' Adam said. 'What can I get for a rib?'

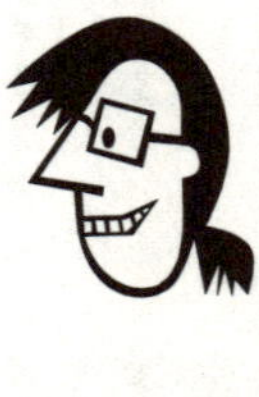

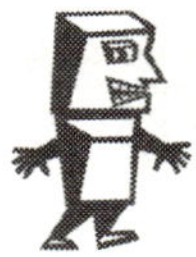

A man comes home to find his wife packing her bags.

'Where are you going?' he asked.

'To London! I found out that there are men that will pay me £200 to do what I do for you for nothing!'

The man thought for a moment, and then began packing his bags.

'What do you think you are doing?' she screamed.

'Going to London with you… I want to see how you live on £400 a year!'

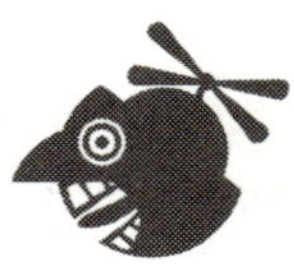

'IF I GIVE YOU A BLOW JOB, WON'T I LOSE YOUR RESPECT?' SAID THE BLONDE.

'NOT AS LONG AS YOU'RE GOOD AT IT.'

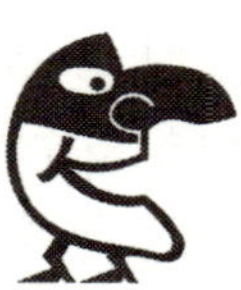

Chemical Analysis

Element: Woman

 Symbol: WO

Discoverer: Adam

Atomic Mass:

Accepted at 53.5kg but known to vary from 40–200kg

Occurrence:

Found wherever man is.
Surplus quantities in all urban areas.

Physical Properties:

Found in various states, ranging from virgin metal to common ore.
Surface often covered in painted film.
Boils at nothing; freezes without known reason.
Melts if given special treatment.
Bitter if incorrectly used.
Non-magnetic but attracted by coins and sport cars.
Yields if pressure applied in the correct places.

Chemical Properties:

Has great affinity for gold, silver and a range of precious stones.
Absorbs great quantities of expensive substances.
May explode spontaneously without prior warning and for no known reason.

Insoluble in liquids, but activity increases greatly by saturation in alcohol.
Most powerful money-reducing agent known to man.

Storage:

Best results are obtained between the ages of 18 and 25 years.

Uses:

Highly ornamental, especially in sports cars.
Can be a great aid to relaxation and a tonic for low spirits.
Very effective cleaning agent.
Can be used on lonely nights as a heating agent (if properly prepared).

Tests:

Pure specimens turn a rosy tint if discovered in raw, natural state.
Turns green if placed besides a better specimen.

Hazards:

Highly explosive in inexperienced hands.
Specimens must be used with great care if experiments are to succeed.
Illegal to possess more then one permanent specimen, although several specimens can be maintained at different locations as long as they do not come into direct contact with each other.

Why is a blonde like a door knob?

Because everybody gets a turn.

What's the mating call of the blonde?

'I'm sooo drunk!'

What's the mating call of the brunette?

'All the blondes have gone home.'

What's the mating call of the redhead?

'Next!'

What are the four types of bra?

The Catholic type supports the masses.

The Salvation Army type lifts the fallen.

The Presbyterian type keeps them staunch and upright.

And the Baptist type makes mountains out of mole hills.

What's the best thing a woman can make for dinner?

Reservations.

What do you do when the dishwasher stops working?

Tell her to get back to work.

Why do women have legs?

So when you're done with them they can leave.

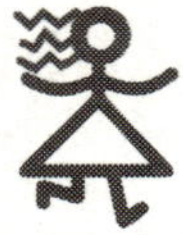

Why did the woman cross the road?

Who cares? What the hell was she doing out of the kitchen?

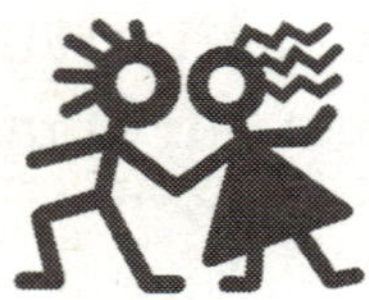

'I think you should learn to garden,' a wife said to her husband, 'then we could do without the gardener.'

'Well if you would learn to fuck me properly,' he replied, 'we could do without the maid.'

A woman was walking through a market and found a beautiful old lamp. Wondering if it might polish up, she rubbed it, and out came a genie.

The genie - as custom would have it - offered her three wishes.

Her first wish was to be powerful, intelligent, and loved by everyone.

The genie thought for a moment, snapped his fingers and turned her into a man.

What do you call a woman with two brain cells?

Pregnant.

Why do women rub their eyes in the morning?

Because they don't have balls.

A successful man is one who makes more money than his wife can spend.

How to talk about women and still be politically correct

She's not a screamer or moaner,
she is vocally appreciative.

She doesn't tease or flirt,
she engages in artificial stimulation.

She's not easy,
she is horizontally accessible.

She is not an airhead,
she is reality impaired.

She does not have a killer body,
she is terminally attractive.

She doesn't have massive boobs,
she is pectorally superior.

She's not dumb,
she's a detour off the information superhighway.

She has not been around,
she's a previously enjoyed companion.

She doesn't get you excited.
She causes temporary blood displacement.

She doesn't get completely ratted,
she gets chemically inconvenienced.

She's not horny,
she is sexually focused.

She's not a slut,
she's a sexual extrovert.

Why is it that ...

men wake up as good-looking as they went to bed.

But women somehow deteriorate during the night.

What's the difference between a woman who smokes a pipe and one who likes S&M?

One likes rough shag and the other likes to shag rough.

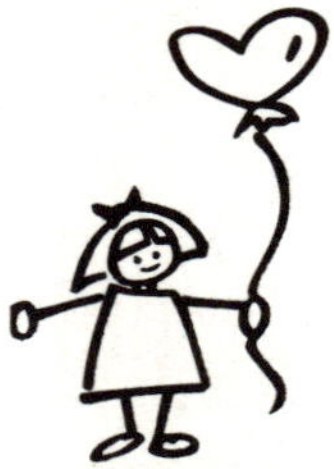

What does a blonde and a beer bottle have in common?

They are both empty from the neck up.

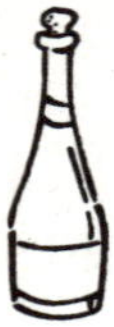

What's the difference between a blonde and the Titanic?

They know how many men went down on the Titanic.

A DOZEN RULES MEN WISH WOMEN KNEW

1 The guy doesn't always have to sleep on the wet spot.

2 Shopping is not a sport.

3 Anyone can buy condoms.

4 Anything you wear is fine. Really.

5 If you really want honesty, don't ask questions you don't want the answers to.

6 Ask for what you want. Subtle hints don't work.

7 The male models with the great bodies you see in magazines are all gay.

8 If something we said can be interpreted two ways, and one of the ways makes you sad or angry, we meant the other one.

9 If we don't look at other women, how can we know how pretty you are?

10 Do not question our sense of direction.

11 When he asks for a threesome with your best friend, he is only joking – unless the answer is yes.

12 Of course, size matters – and boy does he have the grandaddy of them all!

How can you tell which blonde is the waitress?

She's the one with the tampon behind her ear wondering what she did with her pencil.

How can you tell when a blonde is dating?

By the buckle print on her forehead.

What's the difference between a blonde and a sports car?

You don't let your best friend borrow your sports car.

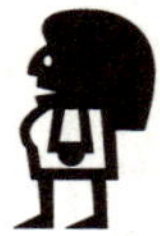

Why did God create Eve?

Because serpents can't bring beer from the fridge.

What do you get when you offer a woman a penny for her thoughts?

Change.

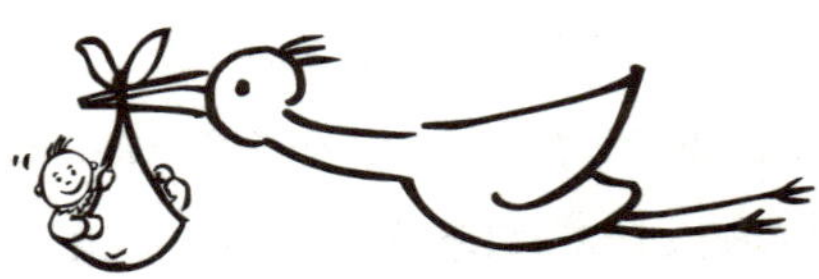

Have you heard about the new birth control pill for men?

You take it the day after and it changes your blood type.

What's the definition of eternity?

The time between you coming and her leaving.

A man found his credit card was stolen but he decided not to report it because the thief was spending less than his wife did.

THE TOP SIX REASONS COMPUTERS MUST BE FEMALE:

1. As soon as you get one, a better one is just around the corner.
2. No one but the creator understands the internal logic.
3. Even your smallest mistakes are committed to memory for future reference.
4. The native language used to communicate with other computers is incomprehensible to everyone else.
5. The message 'Bad Command or File Name' is about as informative as: 'If you don't know why I'm mad at you, then I'm certainly not going to tell you.'
6. As soon as you make a commitment to one, you find yourself spending half of your salary on accessories for it.

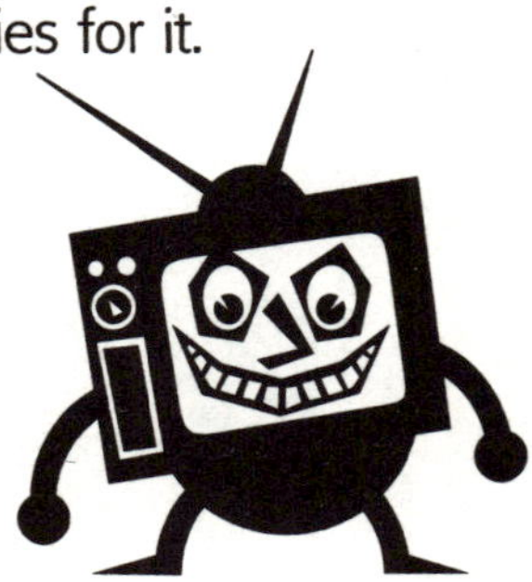

Question: What's the penalty for bigamy?

Answer: Two mothers-in-law

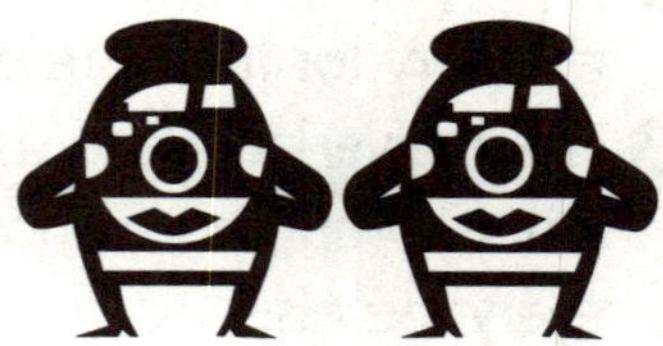

What are the three words you don't want to hear while making love?

'Honey, I'm home!'

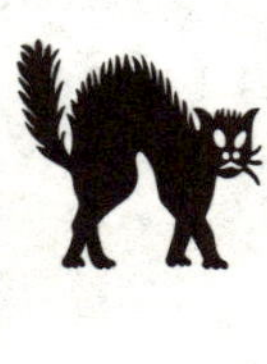

What's the first thing a man invests in when he is planning for his future?

A condom.

My wife is so lazy she even sits down to take a piss.

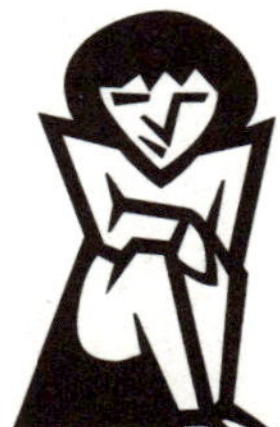

'... and to my wife, Sarah, who always claimed to have a headache when I wanted sex,

I leave all my aspirins.'

Why do women get married in white?

So that they can fit in with the other kitchen appliances.

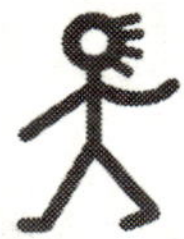

The plural of spouse is spice.

Why did God create man before he created woman?

You always make a rough draft before the final masterpiece.

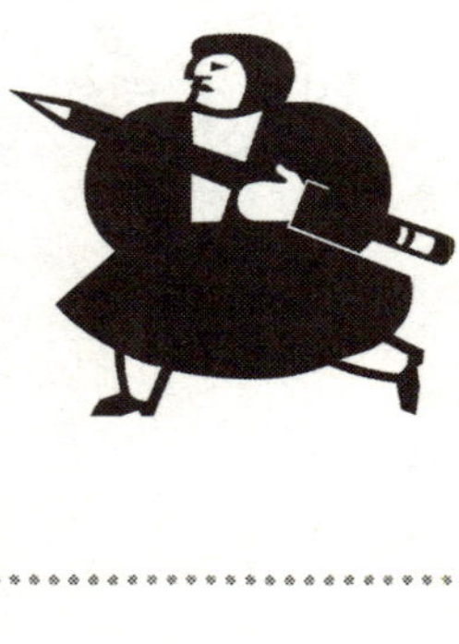

The shortest sentence in the English language is supposed to be: 'I am.'

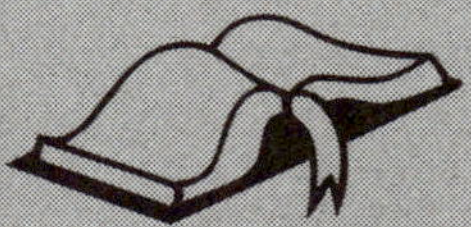

THE LONGEST IS: 'I WILL'

Ten reasons why beer is better than women:

1 When you go to a bar you can always pick up a beer

2 Beer doesn't get jealous when you grab another beer.

3 A beer always goes down easy.

4 You can have more than one beer and not feel guilty.

5 If you pour a beer just right you'll always get good head.

6 You can share a beer with your friends.

7 A frigid beer is a good beer.

8 You always know you're the first one to pop a beer.

9 You can enjoy a beer at any time of the month.

10 Hangovers go away.

THE END